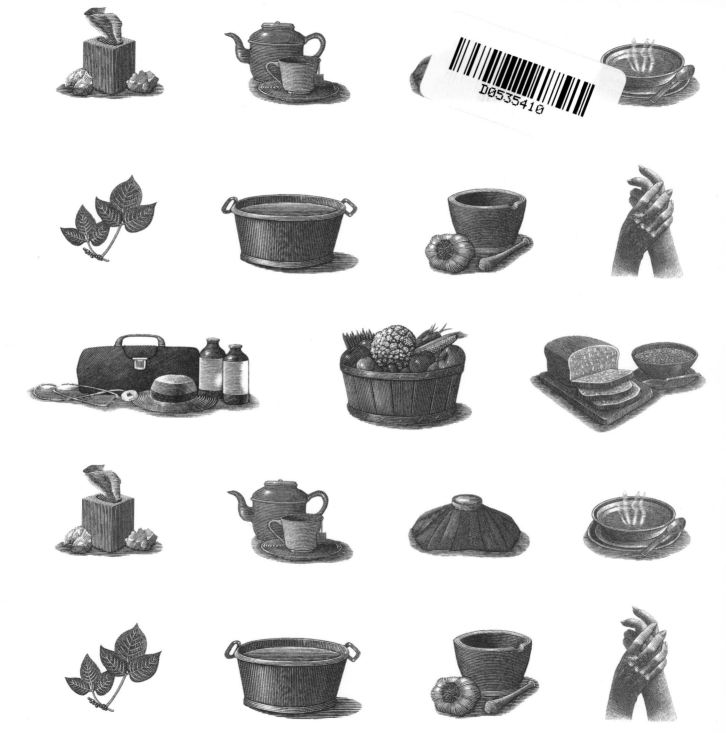

COUNTRY DOCTOR'S
BOOK OF
MEDICAL WISDOM
❧ AND CURES ❧

MICHAEL J. CUMMINGS

CONSULTANT: B. TED BOADWAY, M.D.

PUBLICATIONS INTERNATIONAL, LTD.

Manufactured in U.S.A.

8 7 6 5 4 3 2 1

ISBN: 0-7853-2189-6

NOTICE:
In this book, the authors and editors have done their best to outline the symptoms and general treatment for various conditions, injuries, and diseases. Also, recommendations are made regarding certain drugs, medications, and preparations; and descriptions of certain medical tests and procedures are offered. Different people react to the same treatment, medication, preparation, test, or procedure in different ways. This book does not attempt to answer all questions about all situations that you may encounter.

Neither the Editors of CONSUMER GUIDE® and Publications International, Ltd., nor the consultants, authors, or publisher take responsibility for any possible consequences from any treatment, procedure, test, action, or application of medication or preparation by any person reading or following the information in this book. The publication of this book does not attempt to replace your physician. The authors and the publisher advise the reader to check with a physician before administering any medication or undertaking any course of treatment.

Michael J. Cummings is the author of dozens of health-related articles for various newspapers, magazines, and medical publications. He is a former managing editor of *Grit* and a frequent contributor to *Hospital Benchmarks, Geisinger Medical Center Magazine*, and *FDA Consumer*. Mr. Cummings serves as an adjunct writing instructor at the Pennsylvania College of Technology in Williamsport, Pennsylvania.

B. Ted Boadway, M.D. spent 13 years as a family physician in Thornhill, a suburb of Toronto, before joining the staff of the Ontario Medical Association, where he currently serves as executive director of the Department of Health Policy. He earned his medical degree at the University of Toronto and is a former medical director of Extendicare North York, a 300-bed chronic-care facility. For more than 11 years, Dr. Boadway has been heard regularly on Canadian Broadcasting Corporation national radio programs. He is the author of *Chicken Soup and Other Nostrums*.

Cover Illustration: Robert Crawford
Illustrations: Steven Noble

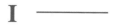 CONTENTS

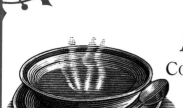
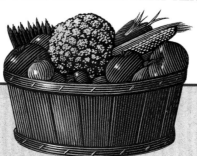

AT-HOME HEALING

If you're like most folks, you probably spend only one to five hours a year in your physician's office and maybe a couple of hours more visiting your dentist. The rest of the time, you probably tend to your health needs yourself.

Got a backache? Are you tense or depressed? What's the best way to treat a headache, a sunburn, or a nosebleed? *Country Doctor's Book of Medical Wisdom and Cures* offers doctor-approved lifestyle strategies and timeless home remedies you can use safely and effectively—for everything from colds and constipation to urinary tract infections.

If you're among those who smoke, if you drink too much, eat a diet high in fat, or succumb too readily to the comforts of an easy chair over the invigorating demands of a walk or bike ride, you will declare yourself open prey for the great killer afflictions of our time: heart disease and cancer. If you need to walk away from an unhealthy lifestyle—and leave behind a trail of bad habits—use this book to form the foundation on which to build your wellness program. You'll find sensible advice about nutrition, exercise, stress reduction, addiction avoidance, and coping with depression. Follow these words of wisdom and you'll be taking an important step toward gaining control of your lifestyle and making the right health choices.

Country Doctor's Book of Medical Wisdom and Cures offers many tried-and-true therapies, including herbal remedies that can be used to treat a migraine or cure a cold and poultices that fight infection. Some of these remedies require little preparation—like cranberry juice, which, according to research, may be effective in preventing bladder infections. Others—like poultices for relieving minor cuts and abrasions—will require more effort: You will need to combine powders or oils with other ingredients before you apply the poultice to your injury.

Like prescription medications, these home remedies may work well for some people and not so well for others. If a particular remedy doesn't seem right for you, check with your doctor before using it—or simply don't use it at all.

Be aware that you should not attempt to treat serious illnesses—or suspected serious illnesses—with the home remedies discussed in this book without first consulting a doctor. Self-treatment may only delay the professional treatment you require and, if the illness worsens, diminish your chances for complete and quick recovery.

As you use *Country Doctor's Book of Medical Wisdom and Cures*, share the information with other members of your family, especially those who could most benefit by it, such as smokers and couch potatoes. Perhaps you'll even decide to launch a wellness program together—improving your chances of reaching your wellness goals.

Remember, folks, there is strength in numbers.

LIVING WELL ❧

"**H**abit is habit," Mark Twain wrote, "and not to be flung out the window by any man, but coaxed downstairs a step at a time."

Now is the time to gather up your bad habits, coax them downstairs, and send them packing. More than any medication or hospital machine, it is your lifestyle that plays the biggest role in whether you stay well. Unfortunately, a good many folks refuse to accept that fact.

According to the National Institutes of Health, half of all Americans don't get regular exercise. Eighty percent refuse to eat the right foods. One-third of adults and nearly one-fifth of children are overweight. And sixty million Americans continue to smoke cigarettes.

Obviously these folks need a good talking to. Afflictions caused by unhealthful lifestyles include high blood pressure, heart disease, stroke, lung cancer, emphysema, obesity, cirrhosis of the liver, stress, and depression. It isn't easy to overcome old habits. What it takes is grit, determination, and a positive attitude. You must want to be well. You must choose to be well.

This chapter will assist you in your wellness efforts by providing useful information and advice about smoking, alcohol abuse, nutrition, exercise, and stress management.

SMOKING AND ALCOHOL ABUSE

According to author Alvin Schwartz, there was once a town so healthy they had to shoot somebody to start a cemetery.

It's a safe bet that nobody in that town—wherever it was—drank to excess or smoked cigarettes. Smoking and drinking are, after all, the twin terrors of medicine. In terms of illness, family problems, lost work days, social discord, and death by accident, disease, and suicide, these vices rival the devastation of an all-out war. In fact, cigarettes and alcohol have killed more Americans—dentists, barbers, bellboys, plumbers, waitresses, farmers—than all the wars in America since Columbus' arrival.

Cigarettes alone figure in the deaths of nearly 400,000 Americans every year and in the illness of millions more. If you tend to prefer comparisons, that would be like having the entire population of North and South Dakota die every three years. And no wonder. Among the approximately 300 known poisons in tobacco smoke are arsenic, cyanide, carbon monoxide, and formaldehyde.

Practically everyone knows that cigarettes cause lung cancer. But not everyone is aware that cigarettes also cause cancer of the mouth, larynx, esophagus, stomach, bladder, kidney, blood, and pancreas. Cigarettes also cause high blood pressure, heart disease, stroke, emphysema, and chronic bronchitis. According to research from the Rose Medical Center in Denver, Colorado, a 25-year-old who smokes two packs of cigarettes a day will die 8.3 years sooner than a nonsmoker. Think of what those 8.3 years mean: all the unwritten poems, the unattended family reunions, and the unspoken conversations with your children and grandchildren.

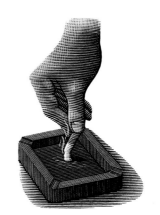

Alcohol abuse is a major cause of violence, suicide, economic ruin, and family turmoil.

But the devastation doesn't end with the smoker. Nonsmokers exposed to secondary smoke at home or at work can develop thickening of the arteries ten percent faster than unexposed non-smokers, according to a study of 8,415 people by the Bowman Gray School of Medicine in Winston-Salem, North Carolina. Children of smokers are among the most frequent victims of secondary smoke: They suffer more respiratory problems and miss more school days than children of nonsmokers.

Another hazard to society's well being is alcohol abuse. Alcohol abuse is a major cause of violence, suicide, economic ruin, and family turmoil. It contributes to the deaths of 100,000 Americans every year from alcohol-related forms of cancer, heart disease, liver disease, and other illnesses. In addition, it kills or injures thousands more in alcohol-related motor-vehicle accidents. An organization called Mothers Against Drunk Driving (MADD) provides the following grim statistics:

Some 16,589 persons died in alcohol-related traffic accidents in 1994, accounting for 40.8 percent of all traffic fatalities. In that same year, one million people suffered injuries in alcohol-related traffic accidents. Two of every five Americans will be involved in an alcohol-related motor-vehicle accident at some time in their lives unless remedial action is taken.

If you're among those who smoke cigarettes or drink alcohol to excess, tell your physician. Your doctor can support and advise you as you struggle with your habit—and point you in the right direction when you decide to give it up. The good news is that quitting your habit can instantly improve your well being. In many cases, your body immediately begins to repair the damage that has been done: Within 15 years, an ex-smoker's risk of suffering a heart attack will be about the same as a nonsmoker's.

No, quitting is not easy. But it is well within everyone's capability, as millions of former smokers and problem drinkers have proved. Begin by admitting you have a problem. Then—with the assistance of relatives, friends, and your physician—determine why you continue to support your bad habits. For example, do you smoke or drink to relieve tension? If so, ask yourself what's causing the tension. Tight deadlines at work? Money problems? Feelings of social inadequacy? (Many people light up cigarettes in social situations to have "something to do with their hands." Some people drink to excess to lower their inhibitions.)

Once you know what's behind your habit, you can begin working on eliminating its cause. When properly motivated, some smokers can quit cold turkey. Others find it helpful to join a support group, seek counseling, or enroll in a smoking-cessation program.

University of Texas researchers have found that "scheduled smoking" can help people quit. Here's how it works: When cutting down, you decide to smoke only at certain times—say 8 a.m., 2 p.m., and 8 p.m. In doing so, you reduce the effects of subtle smoking prompts such as coffee, food, stress, and fatigue. Eventually the prompts lose their effect, making it easier to quit smoking altogether. One year after a scheduled-smoking study, researchers said 44 percent of the people who "quit by the clock" remained nonsmokers, compared with 22 percent who quit cold-turkey and 18 percent who quit in other ways.

One aid that has come along in recent years is the transdermal nicotine patch, now available at drug stores without a doctor's prescription. This device is a tiny decal the user sticks to the skin. During the day the patch releases nicotine into the body, satisfying the smoker's physical need for the drug. Over a period of weeks or months, the dosage released gradually declines, weaning the user off nicotine. Studies have shown that the success rate of the transdermal nicotine patch doubles when the user couples the program with participation in a support group.

Unfortunately, there's no "alcohol patch" for problem drinkers. And cutting down gradually on your own just won't work, because one small portion of alcohol inevitably leads to another—and another, and another.

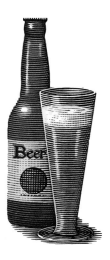

If you're a short-term problem drinker, you may not require hospitalization or other extraordinary measures, but you surely will need the help of others. Many problem-drinkers have found the organization Alcoholics Anonymous to be a very effective program. (AA members include not only short-term problem drinkers but also alcoholics who have "dried out" at detoxification clinics.) At AA meetings, alcohol abusers share their experiences and receive psychological support. Through AA's famous Twelve Step program, members learn to abstain one day at a time. There are no fees. There are no special requirements to join.

Drugs are also available to help ease the transition to sobriety. One of them, Antabuse, makes you sick whenever you drink. Other drugs make the effects of alcohol less pronounced and, therefore, less pleasurable.

Recognizing that alcohol abuse is a problem for the people around the drinker, not just the drinker alone, AA also operates Al-Anon for family members and Alateen for teenage children of alcoholics. In such groups relatives not only learn how to cope in their environment, but they can also learn how to support the alcoholic during the difficult recovery period.

If an underlying psychological problem caused you to begin drinking in the first place, or if a psychological problem arose while you were drinking, you may also need to undergo counseling as you adjust to your new, healthier lifestyle.

Once you kick your addiction—whether it's tobacco or alcohol—you will experience an urge to resume your habit from time to time. But those feelings will lessen over time as new, more productive activities occupy your energies, and new routines and patterns replace the old.

Problem drinkers may need to undergo counseling as they adjust to a new, healthier lifestyle.

EATING WELL

One day experts say it's okay to eat eggs. The next day they say it's not. Milk is good for you, we hear, because it contains calcium and builds strong bones. Milk is bad for you, we hear, because it contains too much artery-clogging saturated fat. So who do you believe?

There's probably a little bit of truth in much of what you read and hear. But there's a lot of truth in what the Greeks advised centuries ago: "All things in moderation, nothing in excess." To that, we should add the following commonsense principles:

1. Tailor your diet to your medical history.

No two people are the same. Their blood pressure, cholesterol level, and metabolic rate differ. Therefore, because you are different, it's best to learn all you can about your body before you develop a plan to improve your diet. If a physical exam reveals you have high blood pressure, for example, you will have to cut down on salty foods—and remove the salt shaker from the table. If you're allergic to milk, which is rich in calcium, you'll have to place other calcium-rich foods on your menu. If you're frequently tense or anxious, you may have to avoid caffeinated products. Talk with your physician. The more you know about your nutritional needs, the better you will be able to fulfill them.

2. Eat a variety of foods.

From time to time, most of us indulge in a hearty meal of meat and potatoes. But if you eat meat and potatoes every noon and night, you won't get the variety of nutrients your body needs. Eventually you could develop a nutritional deficiency that could lead to illness. For example, a calcium deficiency can result in the bone-weakening disease osteoporosis. Iron deficiency can lead to the fatiguing condition known as anemia. And a deficiency in B-complex vitamins can lead to nervousness and nausea. Some of the more than 100 symptoms or conditions caused by or associated with vitamin and mineral deficiencies include muscle weakness, insomnia, depression, diarrhea, constipation, dizziness, headache, apathy, dry skin, itching, trembling, numbness, irritability, and loss of appetite.

Which foods should you eat and in what amounts?

First, make fruits, vegetables, grains, and legumes the mainstay of your diet, accounting for 55 to 60 percent of your total calorie intake. In its dietary guidelines, the U.S Department of Agriculture (USDA) recommends that you eat 6 to 11 servings of grain products a day, 3 to 5 servings of vegetables and legumes, and 2 to 4 servings of fruit. These foods are generally very low in fat and very high in essential nutrients. Besides providing the vitamins, minerals, amino acids, and other nutrients you need to remain healthy, they also are an excellent source of fiber, or roughage. This coarse, stringy substance not only helps cleanse your body of excess fat and cholesterol and promotes regular bowel movements, but it also appears to reduce your risk of developing colon cancer and other intestinal diseases. An excellent source of fiber is breakfast cereal; look for the fiber content listing on the side of the box. Salads, vegetables, and wholegrain breads are also good sources of fiber.

Second, eat moderate amounts of foods in the meat group (red meat, poultry, fish, eggs, and nuts) and the

Make fruits, vegetables, grains, and legumes the mainstay of your diet.

milk group (milk, cheese, yogurt, and other dairy products). According to the USDA, two to three servings a day from each group will meet your nutritional needs. Moderation is necessary because many foods in these groups contain high amounts of saturated fat and cholesterol, which can contribute to the development of heart disease and other illnesses. (A diet high in saturated fats—including those animal fats found in butter and meats—has been found to increase the serum cholesterol level in the blood and, therefore, increase the risk of developing atherosclerosis. Less saturated fats, such as those found in olive oil, canola oil, and the oils in some fish and nuts, are better dietary choices. Not only are they tasty and great to use in cooking, but they're also very nutritious.)

Although the foods found in both the meat and milk groups are excellent sources of protein—which is vital to building and maintaining organs, muscles, cartilage, and skin—your body doesn't require large amounts of protein. According to standards set by the Food and Nutrition Board of the National Academy of Sciences, a 150-pound person requires about 66 grams of protein a day. A four-ounce hamburger alone will meet half that requirement. What if you eat more protein than you need? If you're healthy, the extra protein probably will be converted to sugar. It's the saturated fat and cholesterol found in most protein-containing foods that should concern you— they may remain in the body as excess fat, potentially causing serious health problems.

3. Eat only the number of calories your body needs.

It's not how many calories you consume that matters. It's whether you use those calories. If you're an Olympic swimmer, a lumberjack, or a letter carrier you require more calories than the average person because you expend more calories. It's simple arithmetic. However, if you take in 3,500 calories a day but use only 2,500, your body will store the extra calories as fat. If you make a habit of piling up fat, you'll gain weight. And if you exceed your recommended weight by 20 or 30 pounds—that is, if you become obese—you'll increase your risk of developing a range of diseases. In recent years, Americans have, in fact, been piling up fat. According to the USDA, between 1991 and 1994, the average American gained 11 pounds.

Obesity is the leading cause of diabetes in the United States, according to Michael D. Myers, M.D., a specialist in eating and weight disorders in Los Alamitos, California. But the risks don't stop there. Obesity can also significantly increase the risk of developing high blood pressure, heart disease, degenerative arthritis, gallstones, and cancer. And, Myers says, obese women may have triple the risk of developing cancer of the breast, uterus, cervix, and ovaries.

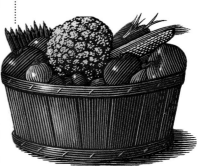

So how many calories does the average person need? Victor Herbert, M.D., a professor at the Mount Sinai School of Medicine in New York, says an average "sedentary adult" requires about 10 calories for each pound of weight to perform basic functions such as breathing, digesting food, and circulating blood. In addition, this sedentary adult requires 3 calories for each pound of weight to carry out routine daily activities, such as walking, eating, or driving a car. Thus, a 175-pound sedentary man would need 2,275 calories a day (175×10 plus 175×3). If this man decided to take up tennis, expending an additional 500 calories each day, then he would need 2,775 calories a day (2,275 + 500).

4. Limit your intake of fat.

Fat makes food taste good. And a certain amount of it is essential to provide energy and enable the body to absorb vitamins A, D, E, and K. You will find an abundance of fat in sausage, most red meats, bacon, salad dressings, deep-fried battered foods, potato chips, ice cream—practically anything that's greasy or creamy. Unfortunately, fat promotes weight gain. (One gram of fat contains 9 calories; one gram of protein or carbohydrates contains only 4 calories). And weight gain can lead to a variety of serious health problems.

The worst kind of fat is saturated fat. It causes the body to produce excessive amounts of cholesterol. Cholesterol that's deposited in your arteries is known as plaque. Over time, these plaques may grow larger and larger. Blood platelets that circulate through your body to aid in clotting sometimes stick to plaque deposits, making them grow all the faster. Eventually, a plaque deposit can grow so large that it cuts off the flow of blood and its life-giving oxygen. When that hap-

As a rule, try to stick with foods that are low in saturated fat.

pens, you could suffer a heart attack or stroke. As a rule, try to stick with foods that are low in saturated fat. Generally, no more than 30 percent of your calories should come from fats, and no more than 10 percent should come from saturated fats.

5. Limit your cholesterol intake.

Cholesterol helps your body produce bile acids, cell membranes, sex hormones, and the protective covering of nerves called myelin. Interestingly, your body produces just about all the cholesterol it needs. Therefore, the cholesterol you get from food is overkill. And if you continually overload your body with cholesterol, you put your arteries at risk of becoming clogged with plaque.

Among the foods high in cholesterol are organ meats, eggs, desserts, and many of the foods that are high in saturated fat. As a general rule, you should limit your intake of cholesterol to no more than 300 milligrams a day.

6. Go easy on salt.

Salt consists of 40 percent sodium and 60 percent chloride. The sodium in salt is vital to maintaining your body's fluid balance and blood pressure. You couldn't live without sodium. The trouble is, as with cholesterol, a little bit of sodium goes a long way. In fact, you need only about 500 milligrams of sodium a day, roughly the amount contained in one-fifth of a teaspoon of salt.

The maximum intake of sodium should not exceed 2,400 milligrams a day, or about a teaspoon of salt, according to U.S.

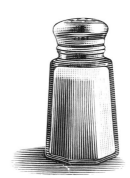

government guidelines. Among foods high in sodium content are bacon, ham, smoked fish, corned beef, pickles, olives, frozen dinners, salad dressings, and practically all canned and processed foods. (Fresh foods usually contain little or no sodium.)

To monitor your sodium intake, read disclosure labels on cartons, packages, and cans, then mark down the amount of sodium you consume when you eat a serving of food. For example, if you eat a serving of bean soup for lunch, you would mark down the amount of sodium in one serving—about 800 milligrams. That would mean you could consume 1,600 more milligrams of sodium during the day before reaching the maximum recommended intake of 2,400 milligrams.

7. Go easy on sugar.

Table sugar, or sucrose, is only one of many kinds of sugar. Other varieties occur naturally in foods. The sugar lactose occurs in milk, and the sugar maltose occurs in the malt in beer. Fruit contains a very sweet sugar called fructose; it also contains the sugars sucrose and glucose.

Your body manufactures glucose from the fruit, vegetables, grains, and other carbohydrates you eat. Glucose is important to the body because it provides fuel and maintains the proper functioning of cells. However, because the body can make or acquire all the glucose it needs from natural foods, you don't need to add glucose—or any other kinds of sugars—to the foods you eat.

KEEPING FIT

When Anne Clarke, of Carol Stream, Illinois, ran a series of footraces in the late 1980s, she sometimes had to compete against younger runners—people who were in their sixties or early seventies. "But I still managed to win 40 national awards," she said. She turned 80 in 1989.

Clarke, a retired teacher, would run five to seven miles a day to stay fit and to train for local, national, and international events, including 10-kilometer races. No doubt some onlookers may have wondered if that sort of vigorous exercise was really safe for older folks.

The fact is, everyone in every age group who is generally healthy and physically able should exercise vigorously—and often. Karl F. Hempel, M.D., a family physician in Tallahassee, Florida, and a diplomate of the American Board of Family Practice, says, according to new government guidelines, everyone should exercise at least 30 minutes a day seven days a week. (But the daily exercise can be cumulative: Two 15-minute exercise periods—or three 10-minute periods—will meet the day's recommended 30-minute requirement.)

What's so good about exercise? Well, besides enabling you to run races, it also:

- Reduces your risk of developing high blood pressure
- Lowers your blood pressure if your pressure is already too high

- Decreases your risk of developing heart disease
- Improves your survivability if you have heart disease
- Enables you to control your weight
- Strengthens your muscles
- Maintains your bone density
- Reduces tension and anxiety
- Improves your physical appearance

Must you run races or climb mountains to stay in shape? Not at all. Americans who don't regularly exercise can achieve cardiovascular fitness simply by walking, riding a bike, or even dancing. Cardiovascular fitness refers to the body's ability to deliver and process oxygen at optimum levels. In other words, if you are cardiovascularly fit, your heart will pump more oxygen per beat, and you will have more endurance. With regular vigorous exercise, your heart will become stronger and stronger, and it will be able to meet demands more efficiently.

Activities that build cardiovascular fitness are called aerobic exercises because they cause sustained heavy breathing. Swimming, skiing, and skipping rope are all aerobic activities. If you regularly exercise aerobically, you can achieve a high level of cardiovascular fitness. Activities that keep you in motion produce better results than activities that make you stop and start repeatedly. For example, although playing golf is good exercise, it does not require a long period of sustained exertion. You walk, then stop; you walk, then stop. Jogging and roller-skating, on the other hand, keep you moving constantly, giving your heart a good workout. (There are also some good old-fashioned exercises that can boost cardiovascular fitness, including pitching hay, pulling weeds, and digging post holes. Just don't stop to gossip with the neighbors for too long.)

Besides aerobic exercise, it's a good idea to include in your regimen exercises that increase muscle strength and flexibility. The stronger and more flexible you are, the less likely you will be to pull a muscle, tear a ligament, throw out your back, or break a bone. Push-ups are an excellent exercise to improve upper body strength. And stretching exercises will increase your overall muscle elasticity, enabling you to bend, turn, and pivot with less risk of injury.

Before you start a vigorous exercise program, you should have a physical exam. For middle-aged and older folks, this examination should include a stress test designed to detect heart problems. The test is relatively simple. While you walk or run on a treadmill, monitors attached to your chest measure your heart activity as well as your blood pressure and pulse.

After receiving your physician's okay, choose one or more activities you are likely to enjoy and stick with them. If they require special equipment—such as running shoes for jogging or a protective helmet for biking—be sure to select comfortable, high-quality products.

Precede each of your workouts with a warm-up period that gradually elevates the heart rate and increases the flow of oxygen-rich blood to the muscles. Five to ten minutes of moderate

Before you start a vigorous exercise program, you should have a physical exam.

activity, such as stretching your arms and your legs, is usually a sufficient warm-up period.

At the end of your workout, don't stop abruptly. Instead cool down by gradually slowing your activity. Cooldowns help prevent a sudden drop in blood pressure. Moreover, they reduce the likelihood that you will become stiff and sore after your workout.

During the first few weeks of your exercise program, don't try to reach all of your exercise goals at once. Instead, break yourself in gradually. For example, if brisk walking is your choice of exercise, you might consider limiting yourself to a half-mile or so early on, then increase your distance to a mile and beyond. Trying to accomplish workout goals too quickly can result in serious injury: Remember, you're in it for the long haul. If at any time you sense that you are overtaxing yourself, it's probably a sign you *are* trying to do too much too soon. If exercise causes chest pain, faintness, dizziness, or weakness, or it causes you to gasp for air, stop your activity immediately and pay a visit to your physician.

If you live in an area where severe weather conditions keep you indoors in the winter or summer, consider investing in exercise equipment, such as treadmills, rowing machines, aerobic riders, and exercise bikes. The more sophisticated machines can monitor your heart rate and keep a daily record of your activities. Of course, you can turn the weather to your advantage, too. In the winter, you can ski or ice-skate. In the summer, try swimming or go canoeing.

Whatever exercise you do—and wherever you do it—the important thing is to keep doing it. Continuing your exercise program will help you live a longer, healthier life.

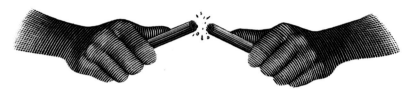

MANAGING STRESS

Stress comes in two varieties: good and bad. Although the two are very different, both varieties may quicken the heartbeat, raise the blood pressure, tense the muscles, and increase the flow of perspiration.

Good stress energizes us to meet the challenge of the moment. It enables a 110-pound mother to defend her child against an attacking dog, a firefighter to enter a burning building to save an elderly man, and a mountain climber to call up hidden reserves of strength to reach the summit.

Bad stress saps energy by making us respond to a situation, or stressor, with anger, crankiness, frustration, disappointment, worry, irritability, and other negative emotions. If you've ever queued up in the 10-items-or-less-line at the supermarket only to discover that everybody in front of you has 50 items or more, you know the meaning of bad stress. Supermarket lines are only one

Nicotine and caffeine can jangle your nerves and make you irritable.

of the many stressors people face every day. (Other stressors include unreasonable deadlines, unreasonable workloads, an uncertain job future, traffic congestion, noisy neighbors, crime, pollution, balancing the checkbook, marital problems, and single parenthood.)

Many stressors are unique to our age. Take caregiving, for example. Thanks to medical and technological advancements, the life expectancy of the average American has increased about 30 years since the horse-and-buggy days. However, because not all elderly Americans are capable of independent living, the task of caring for them usually falls to their sons and daughters. And if the sons and daughters have their own children to raise, they end up doing triple duty—as workers, parents, and caregivers.

If you suffer from stress that's accompanied by such symptoms as headaches, palpitations, insomnia, appetite loss, and anxiety, you should see your physician. However, if you're like most of us, you simply need to get a better grip on your lifestyle. Here's how:

- Avoid nicotine and caffeine. They can jangle your nerves and make you irritable.
- Avoid resorting to alcohol to relieve tension. Alcohol is a depressant and will only make you feel worse in the long run.
- Treat yourself to an occasional relaxing massage.
- If you have an elderly loved one to care for, don't try to do everything yourself. Instead, take advantage of community nursing services or day-care centers for the elderly. You may

be eligible for financial assistance. Another option is to ask relatives to spell you on occasion by taking the elderly person in for a week, or perhaps a weekend.

- Learn to laugh at yourself and see the humorous side of life. Play practical jokes, rent a funny movie, and dress up in silly costumes on Halloween.
- Educate yourself about stress-reduction techniques such as meditation and deep-breathing exercises.
- If minor annoyances—such as loud music and waiting in long lines at the supermarket—stress you, try to figure out a way around them. If junior likes to listen to heavy metal music in the next room, buy him a pair of headphones for his birthday. If you want to avoid waiting in long lines at the supermarket, shop during off-hours. If you can't handle the traffic congestion, take a different, scenic route home.
- In addition to your yearly two- or three-week vacation, take occasional weekend vacations. If you have children, go on picnics, take hikes, or visit amusement parks.

Of course, some stressors in life—such as the IRS, inclement weather, congenital illness, and death—are beyond your control. So, rather than focusing on events you cannot change, focus instead on events you can. Begin by taping a copy of Reinhold Niebuhr's famous admonition to your refrigerator:

"God grant us grace to accept with serenity the things that cannot be changed, courage to change the things which should be changed, and the wisdom to distinguish the one from the other."

> **Rather than focusing on events you cannot change, focus instead on events you can.**

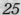

PEACEFUL LIVING

To country folk, one of the best remedies for afflictions of the spirit is the fishing pole. If you take one in hand and sneak off to a stream that nobody knows about, you'll catch a whole passel of peace and contentment, to say nothing of a trout or two.

"God never did make a more calm, quiet, innocent recreation than angling," Izaak Walton wrote more than three centuries ago. It's a fair bet that many a country doctor before and since Walton has prescribed the fishing remedy to harried patients. The hiking remedy isn't bad either. All you need to do is put on a pair of sturdy shoes and head off to a patch of woods, preferably where moss carpets the earth and the smell of pine scents the air.

It's pleasurable escapes such as these—little vacations from the daily grind—that help many people prevent the molehills of distress they face every day from growing into mountains of anguish. Who, after all, can be tense when he's face to face with a chipmunk or taking an impromptu nap in the shade of tall sycamores, birches, and hemlocks.

Peace and contentment. They're as precious to our minds as good health is to our bodies.

But how do you achieve peace and contentment when there are so many forces working against you in this fast-paced, survival-of-the-fittest world? What should you do if your mental pain hangs on, leechlike, in spite of your best efforts—fishing trips, hiking excursions, and a dozen and one other remedies?

THINKING POSITIVELY

Stress breeds negative thinking. Negative thinking breeds stress. It's a vicious circle. But it doesn't have to be that way. If you begin to see the good side of things—if you can laugh and enjoy life again—your positive thinking can help chase away stress and restore peace of mind.

Today doctors realize that a positive attitude can be a crucial factor in overcoming mental and physical illness of every kind, because a positive attitude helps mobilize the healing forces within the body. So, if you are now struggling with major stress, don't overlook the power within you to fight back. It can be a potent weapon.

EXERCISING VIGOROUSLY

When you're under stress, the tension that builds remains inside you, much as steam remains in a tightly covered pot of boiling water. However, if you exercise, you give your body a way to release that pent-up tension and energy. If your exercise is vigorous and sustained, you may be able to achieve a heightened sense of well-being. Here's why: When you exercise vigorously—for example, if you ride a bike or walk for a half hour—your pituitary gland secretes feel-good hormones called endorphins that actually help to raise your spirits. Some good stress-busting activities to consider include walking, jogging, swimming, bicycling, skiing, and dancing.

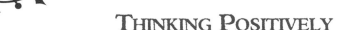

MAINTAINING NUTRITION

When there's a small war going on inside you, you need a steady supply of ammunition—that is, nutritious food—to hold your own. Although your appetite may fall off, you should not skip meals or live on junk food. Doing so can result in nutritional deficiencies and make you more vulnerable to all sorts of illnesses. Also, don't gorge on food to smother your stress. Doing so can result in stomach distress and perhaps an entirely new problem: weight gain.

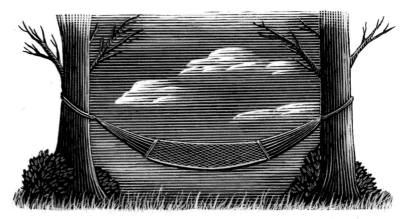

GETTING ENOUGH REST

Sleep deprivation can aggravate the stress you're under, whatever the cause, resulting in impaired concentration, forgetfulness, and irritability. In addition, it can increase your likelihood of having an accident or developing an illness.

In other words, inadequate sleep can spell big trouble. How much sleep is the right amount? That depends on the individual. Some people need only six hours of sleep each night while others need eight to ten hours. Your body will tell you whether you need more or less. If you're under a lot of stress, don't be surprised if you feel more tired than usual. During stressful times, your body may require additional hours of sleep.

USING RELAXATION TECHNIQUES

Most of us wouldn't describe a warm bath or a walk in the park as a "relaxation technique." But that's exactly what these activities are. In fact, anything that calms our spirit—smelling a rose, listening to Chopin, walking the dog, viewing a sunset—is a relaxation technique. The following relaxation exercise is a bit more elaborate, but research has proven it to be very effective in countering stress.

Progressive muscle relaxation is a technique that alleviates stress and muscle tension and leaves you feeling relaxed and refreshed. This exercise involves first tensing your muscles, then slowly relaxing them. (Eventually, with repeated use of the technique, you may be able to recognize and relieve muscle tension without having to tense your muscles.) Here are the steps to take:

1. Lie down in a quiet place and close your eyes.
2. Tense your lips by pursing them. Hold the position for five seconds, then relax your lips.

> During stressful times, your body may require additional hours of sleep.

3. Tense your forehead, facial, and neck muscles, maintaining the tension for 5 seconds each time. Relax.

4. Proceed downward, alternately tensing and relaxing different muscle groups. Continue until you have tensed and relaxed all of your muscles, including those in your toes.

SEEKING COUNSEL

If you don't respond to self-help therapies—or if your stress is severe—your doctor may recommend that you see a psychiatrist or other therapist. Some people resist this option. Seeing a "shrink," they believe, will stigmatize them as weak. Actually, seeking professional help is a sign of strength; it demonstrates that you are ready to attack a problem head-on.

The psychiatrist will take a medical history and evaluate your symptoms. Then he will help you identify the cause of your distress. The psychiatrist may offer immediate short-term relief in the form of medication, although drug therapy isn't always necessary. The doctor will also help you develop a long-term solution that focuses on lifestyle adjustments.

BATTLING DEPRESSION

What if you suffer from sadness that is intense and severe—it's not simply the blues? What if your sadness is continuous and unrelenting and you feel dejected, worthless, and hopelessly alone? Then you may be suffering from clinical depression, a condition that is not to be fooled with.

Clinical depression can develop in reaction to the major stressors that will afflict many of us at some point in our lives: the death of a spouse, the death of a close relative, divorce, separation, financial loss, loss of employment, retirement, health problems, sexual problems, and lifestyle changes. In addition, clinical depression can occur as a result of chemical imbalances in the body. Scientists now believe that genetic factors may also make certain individuals more susceptible to experiencing episodes of depression.

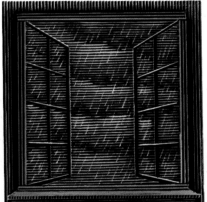

In addition to extreme sadness, victims of depression may develop the following symptoms: loss of interest in life, diminished or increased appetite, insomnia or excessive sleeping, fatigue, constipation, chest pain, achiness, indecision, feelings of guilt over minor matters, and episodes of crying.

If you believe you may be suffering from clinical depression, your first priority should be to see your physician. Because some of the symptoms of depression mimic those of physical illnesses, the doctor will conduct an examination and take a medical history. If the results rule out underlying illnesses and confirm that you have depression, the physician will probably recommend an antidepressant medication that will begin to alleviate your symptoms in two to six weeks. Either the physician will prescribe the medication himself, or he will refer you to a psychiatrist who specializes in treating depression. In addition to drug therapy, your doctor may also recommend cognitive therapy, psychotherapy, or group therapy to help you gain insight into your problems and develop long-term coping skills to deal with difficult times.

As your depression begins to lift, don't assume that the medication will purge you of all daily tension and stress. Like the person you were before you developed depression, you will still react negatively on occasion to stressors such as financial problems and work deadlines—everyone does. But to keep depression at bay, do your best to stay in tip-top mental and physical condition. Eat right. Exercise. Get enough sleep. Avoid tobacco and alcohol. And regularly practice relaxation techniques.

COPING WITH GRIEF

Grief is a part of life. You cannot avoid it and you should not try to. Instead, confront it, and let it run its course. Along the way, do not suppress your feelings. Doing so will only postpone or prolong your grief while intensifying your bottled-up stress.

Initially you may react to the loss of a loved one with shock, disbelief, and profound sadness. Later, you may feel lonely, helpless, and confused. You may even feel anger, wanting to blame someone for the loss, even yourself. Because you are under stress, you may develop palpitations, shortness of breath, insomnia, and other symptoms. Realize, though, that experiencing such symptoms is to be expected during these tough times.

Both men and women should not be afraid to cry. Your tears are paying tribute to the life of the loved one; they are a form of eulogy. And tears provide an outlet for your emotional stress.

Don't be afraid to talk about your feelings. Airing them will help you make sense of the loss and speed your acceptance of it. It will also help you deal with any sense of guilt you may be feeling over some past hurt you may have caused the deceased. Women, it has been said, tend to cope better than men in times of loss because they are quick to seek out the company of a sympathetic listener. If you are a man, take a lesson from the women around you.

Understanding grief and learning how to cope with its emotions can be very difficult. If you believe you need the guidance of a physician or therapist to help you through your grief, don't hesitate to contact one. The loss of a loved one is, after all, a major trauma. Seeking the help of a professional may even be advisable if you are currently coping with other distress, such as an illness or an upsetting lifestyle change.

Bear in mind, however, that grieving doesn't mean that you'll feel gloomy all the time. There is nothing improper or unhealthy about laughing or enjoying leisure activities during a grieving period. Nor is there anything wrong with recalling humorous incidents involving the deceased loved one. In fact, it's simply good therapy to do so.

Stress, depression, and grief will invade our lives. Relief can come swiftly if we reach out for help. Asking for help is a "technique" that isn't often discussed, but it is one that is just as important as other types of treatment. We all need to learn to ask for help; none of us is so self-sufficient as to have all the answers.

Don't be afraid to talk about your feelings.

HEALING WAYS

You're likely to stumble across a variety of remedies for practically everything that ails you in this chapter—from backaches and headaches to insomnia and sunburn. Some recommendations may seem familiar, and some may not. Why not give them a try? Sometimes a simple homespun remedy is all it takes to get you back on your feet again.

BACK PAIN

You heave the saddle up on the horse and—ouch!—there goes your back. It's out again.

Eight of every ten Americans suffer episodes of back pain sometime in their lives. The pain may be mild or moderate, or it may be excruciating, making it difficult to perform even simple everyday tasks like tying your shoes or climbing stairs. Strains, the most common cause of back pain, occur when overworked or under-exercised back muscles are pushed beyond their limits.

CAUSES

Many people experience back pain as they age and their joint tissues deteriorate or shift. Back pain can also be caused by sitting for long periods of time; psychological tension; diseases of the kidneys, heart, lungs, intestinal tract, or reproductive organs; osteoporosis; physical malformations; and being overweight. A slipped disk, muscle sprain, ligament strain, a sudden twisting or turning motion, kidney infection, bone disease, tumor, pregnancy, and menstrual cramps can also be blamed for back pain.

SYMPTOMS

Backaches can occur abruptly after physical activity or may develop slowly. The pain may feel like a sharp jab or a dull ache. Severe back pain may also be accompanied by pain or numbness radiating down one or both legs. Most muscular back pain disappears in a week or two, whereas some aches and pains can last up to two months or more.

REMEDIES

- To help keep inflammation and discomfort to a minimum, apply ice to the strained area within 24 hours of the injury. (A bag of frozen peas makes a great ice pack!) Don't put the ice pack directly on your skin, however. Wrap the bag in a thin towel and place it on the injured area for 20 minutes. Take a 30 minute break, then apply the ice pack again for 20 minutes more.
- If it's been more than 24 hours since you injured your back, apply heat to help relieve muscle spasms, because ice will no longer reduce pain or inflammation. A 20-minute soak in the bathtub may be all it takes to get you on your feet again.
- Exercise as soon as you're able. But don't pitch hay or dig a potato field. And don't lift heavy objects or engage in other activities that may unduly stress the back.
- Sit straight to relieve pressure on your spine and back muscles. If you work at a desk, sit closely to it and use a foot rest to elevate your knees just above your hips.

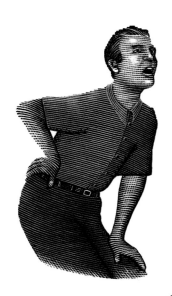

- When sitting, shift position from time to time. Every 30 minutes or so, stand up and walk around or try a stretching exercise. The American Academy of Orthopaedic Surgeons recommends the following exercise for preventing back pain: With your feet several inches apart, place your hands on your lower back and slowly bend backward while keeping your knees straight. Bend back as far as you can and hold your position for a few seconds. Return to your original position. Repeat.
- Sleep on your side on a supportive mattress. Sleeping on your stomach stresses your lower back. When getting out of bed, roll or slide out, rather than "jerking" yourself up.
- Lose weight. Extra weight puts extra strain on back muscles. Sensible, gradual weight loss can help ease back pain.
- Store heavy objects above waist level so you can lift them without stressing your back.
- When lifting an object off the floor, bend your knees without bending your waist. Look straight ahead and keep your shoulders up. If an object feels too heavy, don't try to lift it yourself.

Call your physician if symptoms such as fever, nausea, vomiting, chest pain, dizziness, rapid weight loss, abdominal pain, or sudden bowel or bladder incontinence accompany your back pain; back pain radiates down your leg; or you experience prolonged back pain (lasting for more than one or two weeks).

COLDS

Medical researchers have yet to discover a cure for the common cold. It's no wonder: Any of hundreds of viruses can cause the contagious upper-respiratory infection. Colds generally involve the membranes of the voice box, throat, and nose, but they can also involve the breathing tubes (the trachea and its two branches, called bronchi) leading to the lungs.

CAUSES

Although colds are caused by viruses, your risk of developing a cold is increased by stress, anxiety, fatigue, overwork, smoking, and nutritional problems.

SYMPTOMS

Symptoms of the common cold include coughing, sneezing, hoarseness, nasal and sinus congestion, mild fever, sore throat, fatigue, watery eyes, and loss of appetite.

REMEDIES

- Throw a few extra logs on the fireplace, relax, and get plenty of bed rest.
- Take aspirin or acetaminophen to help relieve body aches and headache. Infants, children, and teenagers should not be given aspirin for a viral infection because of the risk of Reye syndrome, a rare but serious illness reported to be associated with aspirin.

A cure for the common cold has yet to be discovered.

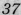

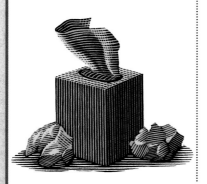

- Take an antihistamine to relieve congestion. Be aware, though, that antihistamines can cause drowsiness. And while decongestants also relieve nasal congestion, they can make you feel jittery and cause insomnia. Some people prefer taking a decongestant during the day and an antihistamine at night.
- Drink plenty of fluids to help thin lung secretions and prevent dehydration. Avoid milk though; in some people, it may thicken lung secretions.
- As part of your fluid therapy, try a traditional remedy that really works—chicken soup. Because it's liquid, it helps prevent dehydration and thins mucus secretions. Because it's hot, it may help promote blood circulation in your throat, speeding healing. Because it contains salt, it may reduce throat swelling. Also, its steamy vapors may help relieve nasal congestion.
- Use a cool-mist vaporizer or take a hot shower to further thin mucus secretions.
- If you're suffering from congestion, apply petroleum jelly to the tip of your nose to relieve chafing and rawness caused by frequent nose blowing.
- Though some scientific evidence suggests otherwise, vitamin C may reduce the severity of your symptoms or the duration of your cold. If you do give it a try, remember to stick to a dosage of no more than 2,000 milligrams a day. Higher doses may cause diarrhea.

Call your physician if you develop white or yellow spots on your throat; you are short of breath; you have a fever that occurs five days after your cold begins; you cough up yellow-green or grayish sputum; you have pain in the chest, ears, or sinuses; or you are unusually lethargic.

CONSTIPATION

For some, regularity means having a bowel movement three times a week; for others, it is part of their daily routine. What matters is not the frequency of your bowel movements, but whether your normal routine alters. Constipation and other changes in bowel habits may be a sign of a serious underlying illness.

CAUSES

Constipation is most commonly caused by a lack of dietary fiber. But stress, failure to drink enough liquids, depression, overuse of laxatives, and adverse reaction to drugs may also be responsible. Possible underlying causes of constipation are kidney disease, cancer, an underactive thyroid gland, tearing of anal tissue, and excessive amounts of calcium in the blood.

SYMPTOMS

Symptoms of constipation include missed bowel movements, straining, hard stools, and sometimes pain and bleeding in the rectal area.

REMEDIES

- Prevent constipation by beginning each day with a high-fiber cereal. Cereals containing 5 grams of fiber or more per serving are best. (Check the side of the cereal box for a complete listing of its contents.)
- Keep up with the fluids. Drink at least eight glasses of water a day.
- Eat plenty of fruits, vegetables, and whole-grain products, which are rich in the fiber you need to promote bowel movements.
- Your diet should include natural laxatives such as prunes, dates, and figs. A commercial product that contains psyllium may also be helpful.
- Allow enough time in your daily schedule for nature to take its course. Go when you feel the urge.
- Exercise vigorously. It'll help speed digested food through the bowels. Walk. Play tennis. Jog.
- Take time to relax. Tension and stress tend to inhibit the bowels from doing their work.
- Keep track of what you eat. If constipation regularly occurs after eating a certain food, try eliminating that food from your diet.

Call your physician if your constipation persists for more than five days; you are unable to pass gas; you bleed during a bowel movement; or you have abdominal cramps or fever.

COUGHING

Coughing is a symptom, not an illness. The cough is a protective reflex: It clears your breathing passages of secretions or irritants such as smoke and dust. As long as it accomplishes this task effectively, coughing should be regarded as a normal and even healthy reaction.

A harsh or forceful cough can be an irritant to the lining of the airways, however. The act of coughing causes the airways to contract. When this happens over and over, it leads to inflamed membranes and helps to perpetuate the cough. Thus, while taking action to relieve your cough, don't ignore its root cause—especially if the cough lasts two weeks or more, if it produces bloody or greenish phlegm, or if it produces no phlegm at all.

CAUSES

Coughing can be caused by colds, flu, bronchitis, pneumonia, emphysema, lung cancer, heart disease, croup, asthma, allergies, postnasal drip, drug reactions, and irritants such as dust, tobacco smoke, and chemical fumes.

SYMPTOMS

Types of coughs include dry coughing that produces little or no phlegm (usually typical of flu and colds); wet coughing that produces phlegm (usually typical of lung infections such as bronchitis and possibly pneumonia); coughing with wheezing (a possible symptom of emphysema); and a barking cough (usually

**Coughing
is a symptom,
not an illness.**

typical of croup, an infection of the vocal cords that occurs in children under age six).

Symptoms that can accompany of a cough include throat soreness, chest pain or burning, feeling of pressure in the chest, and tickle in the throat.

REMEDIES

- If an irritant such as smoke or a chemical is causing your cough, avoid it.
- If an infection such as a cold or the flu is causing your cough, use the home remedies listed in this chapter to help alleviate your symptoms.
- If your cough is wet, drink fluids to soothe your throat and loosen mucus. You may also wish to try a cool-mist vaporizer as well as an over-the-counter cough medication called an expectorant.
- If your cough is dry, drink fluids, especially warm or hot ones, to soothe your throat. You may also want to try a homemade cough syrup of one part lemon juice and two parts honey as well as over-the-counter cough drops that contain the drug dextromethorphan.

Call your physician if you cough up greenish or bloody phlegm; you cough up bright red blood; your cough persists even after your cold or flu disappears; or you experience chest or throat pain or breathing difficulty.

DRY MOUTH

Dry mouth is a condition in which not enough saliva is produced in the mouth. Breathing too much through your mouth—and not enough through your nose—can cause this condition. If your mouth is dry all the time, don't put off remedying the problem. Here's why: Saliva contains an antibacterial agent. When your mouth doesn't get enough of it, the process of tooth decay can increase dramatically. Also, because saliva lubricates the mouth and moistens the food you eat, it makes swallowing easier. Dry mouth can lead to tongue and lip fissures and impair your sense of taste and smell.

CAUSES

Dry mouth may be caused by Sjögren syndrome, diabetes, dehydration, certain medications, and breathing through the mouth.

SYMPTOMS

Symptoms of dry mouth (and sometimes dry throat) include difficulty chewing or swallowing, decreased ability to taste and smell, and tongue and lip fissures.

REMEDIES

- If you have diabetes, drink plenty of water to replace the fluids lost through frequent urination.
- Increase your fluid intake if you are dehydrated as a result of activity or illness.

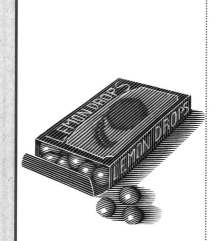

- If a certain medication seems to be leaving your mouth dry, ask your doctor whether a suitable alternative is available.
- If a diet pill seems to be causing the problem, discontinue using it. Instead, try exercising and eating a nutritious, low-calorie diet.
- If a stuffy nose caused by a cold is forcing you to breathe through your mouth, take a hot shower. The steam can help relieve nasal congestion (see Colds, pages 37–39).
- Eat "chewy" meals and snacks to stimulate saliva production. (Grandma's homemade granola bars might be just the ticket to give your mouth the workout it needs.) Between meals, keep your mouth moving with sugar-free gum or a piece of hard candy.

Call your physician if you have symptoms of Sjögren syndrome (dryness of the mucous membranes) or diabetes or you suspect your symptoms are caused by medication you are taking.

FLU

Influenza germs are smart. In order to infiltrate our bodies from year to year, they continually redesign themselves so that no single vaccine can remain effective against them. One year we have the Hong Kong flu. The next year, it's the Leningrad or Taiwan flu. The following year, it's an entirely different strain.

Like a cold, influenza is a contagious upper-respiratory infection, but its symptoms—such as fever and cough—are more distressing. Usually it takes one to two weeks for the illness to run its course and for you to start feeling like yourself again.

CAUSES

The flu is caused by a viral infection. Your risk of getting the flu increases if you suffer from stress or fatigue, if your diet is poor, or if another illness has weakened your immune system.

SYMPTOMS

Flu symptoms include chills, fever, headache, runny nose, muscle aches, hoarseness, sore throat, and dry cough.

REMEDIES

- Get plenty of bed rest.
- Drink plenty of liquids and eat chicken soup to help thin lung secretions and prevent dehydration.
- Avoid milk. It can thicken lung secretions in some people.
- Use a vaporizer to ease congestion.
- Take a pain reliever to help alleviate headache and muscle aches and pains. Children and teenagers should not be given aspirin for a viral illness because of the risk of Reye syndrome, a rare but serious illness reported to be associated with aspirin.
- Gargle with salt water (1 teaspoon salt to a pint of water) to soothe a sore throat. Gargling with strong tea may also help ease throat pain.

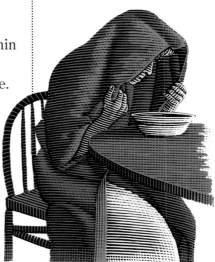

- Use over-the-counter cough syrups, decongestants, and nasal sprays. Be aware that such medications can mask symptoms, however, so don't overexert yourself before you're really recovered.
- Don't smoke. Smoking will only worsen coughing.

Call your physician if your fever or cough worsens; you cough up blood or greenish or yellowish sputum; you are short of breath or have chest pain; or you have other unusual or worrisome symptoms.

HEADACHES

Headache pain may occur in one part of the head or all over the head. One of the most common causes of headaches is tightening of the muscles of the scalp, neck, face, and jaw. Stress and anxiety can trigger this response.

Serious underlying problems, such as a brain tumor or chronic high blood pressure, can also cause headaches. You should see a physician if you suffer from migraines or frequent or unexplained headaches.

CAUSES

Headache pain can be caused by stress, anxiety, smoking, excess alcohol or caffeine consumption, caffeine withdrawal, adverse reactions to medications, fever, irregular eating patterns, sleeping problems, fatigue, eyestrain, awkward sitting or lying positions that strain neck muscles, sinus infection, ear infection, toothache, eating meats containing sodium nitrites, hormonal changes, and a rapid rise in blood pressure as a result of anger, sexual excitement, or vigorous activity.

SYMPTOMS

Symptoms of a headache include pain in the front or back of the head, across the scalp, over the temples, or all over the head. The pain sometimes involves the neck and shoulders as well.

REMEDIES

- Take aspirin or acetaminophen to relieve the pain.
- Apply cold or warm compresses to the affected area.
- Massage shoulder and neck muscles.
- Don't smoke.
- Don't drink alcohol.
- Don't chew gum. Gum-chewing tenses muscles; tense muscles, in turn, can cause a headache.
- Stop sitting or lying in positions that strain neck muscles.
- Keep a regular eating pattern and don't skip meals. If you miss or postpone meals, your blood sugar could fall, causing blood vessels in the head to tighten. This condition can lead to a headache.
- Monitor caffeine consumption. If you drink three or four cups of caffeinated coffee each weekday and then don't drink coffee at all on the weekend, you could suffer a caffeine-withdrawal headache. Headaches also result from

drinking too much caffeine. Try to limit yourself to one or two cups of coffee a day—or don't drink caffeine at all.

- Don't strain your eyes. If you wear eyeglasses, see that you have the correct prescription.
- If you suspect a prescription or nonprescription medication is causing your head pain, talk with your physician about taking an alternative medication.

Call your physician if your pain is noticeable only when you bend your neck or move around; your pain resulted from a head injury; your pain has no apparent cause; your headaches are becoming more frequent or more intense; or your headache is accompanied by blurred vision or dizziness.

HEARTBURN

Heartburn is a burning sensation beneath the breastbone that often radiates to the neck and shoulders. The condition is sometimes accompanied by the regurgitation of a sour, bitter material into your throat or mouth. Heartburn is caused by acid reflux, which is the reverse flow of acid from the stomach to the esophagus, or food pipe.

High-fat foods and caffeinated beverages are common causes of heartburn because they relax the ring of muscle at the top of the stomach, called the lower esophageal sphincter. When the sphincter muscle becomes lazy, it allows acidic stomach contents to move back up the esophagus, causing heartburn.

High-fat foods and caffeinated beverages are common causes of heartburn.

CAUSES

Causes of heartburn include foods with a high fat or high acid content; effervescent drinks; aspirin and other drugs; hiatal hernia; and ulceration of the esophagus. Your risk of developing heartburn increases if you smoke, drink to excess, are overweight, are pregnant, or suffer from stress.

SYMPTOMS

Symptoms of heartburn include a burning sensation in the chest or abdomen, belching, bloating, regurgitation of stomach matter into your throat or mouth, and chest pain.

REMEDIES

- Using wood blocks, elevate the head of your bed at least 6 inches. The elevation assists gravity in keeping your stomach acids where they belong.
- Don't overeat and don't lie down after large meals.
- Don't eat anything two to three hours before going to bed.
- Don't smoke. Cigarettes relax the lower esophageal sphincter and predispose you to heartburn.
- Decrease the amount of alcohol, chocolate, fats, and peppermints you consume. These substances may relax the lower esophageal sphincter.
- If you are overweight, shed the extra pounds. A leaner abdomen decreases the pressure on your stomach, which in turn may lessen reflux.

- Take an over-the-counter antacid to relieve occasional heartburn. Also, ask your pharmacist about a new therapy that combines antacids with an over-the-counter anti-ulcer medication to produce long-lasting relief.
- Chew gum. Gum-chewing increases saliva production. Saliva, in turn, neutralizes regurgitated acids.

Call your physician if you develop heartburn three or four times a week; you experience dizziness or shortness of breath; you experience nausea; you vomit blood; or you have difficulty swallowing.

INSOMNIA

Most of us modern folks regard interruptions of sleep as a source of frustration, especially when sleeplessness extends from late-night television to the rooster's morning crow.

Insomnia can result from a long list of causes—the most common of which often stem from stress and anxiety. For many people, insomnia lasts only a day or two. For others, insomnia may seem to last indefinitely.

CAUSES

Causes of insomnia include stress, anxiety, depression, painful illness, shortness of breath, hot weather, noise, irregular work hours, jet lag, smoking, drinking alcoholic or caffeinated beverages, frequent urination, drug reactions, lack of exercise, and an uncomfortable sleeping environment.

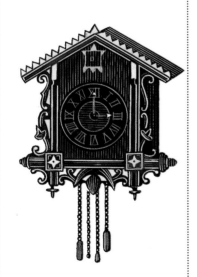

SYMPTOMS

Symptoms of insomnia include irritability, fatigue, and the inability to fall sleep—or stay asleep—at night.

REMEDIES

- Keep regular sleep hours. If a can't-be-missed TV movie happens to start at midnight, program the VCR to record it, and tune into your dreams instead.
- Arise at the same time each morning, even after nights of little sleep. Regular sleeping habits help build successful sleeping patterns in the long run.
- Use relaxation techniques to alleviate stress or anxiety (see Peaceful Living, pages 29–30).
- Make your sleeping environment as comfortable as possible. Plump pillows, a supportive mattress, and cozy sheets and blankets can work wonders.
- Don't smoke. Cravings for nicotine can awaken you several times during the night.
- Don't drink large amounts of any beverage. If you do, it's guaranteed you'll be walking back and forth to the bathroom all night long.
- Limit your alcohol intake or, better yet, avoid alcohol. After its initial calming effect wears off, an alcoholic beverage tends to awaken—and reawaken—you.
- Avoid eating right before going to bed. Your whole body needs to go to sleep, including your stomach.

- Get plenty of exercise during the day or early evening. When bedtime arrives, your body will be ready for sleep.
- Read a book or listen to relaxing music just before going to bed. Reading can make your eyelids heavy; music can calm your spirit.
- If you are tossing and turning, do not try to force sleep; get up. While you're awake, relax: Read a book, work a crossword puzzle, or write a letter. When you're too tired to stay awake, go back to bed and try to sleep again.

Call your physician if your insomnia may be due to depression, stress, or anxiety; you suspect your insomnia is a reaction to a medication you're taking; or your insomnia becomes chronic.

NOSEBLEEDS

Let's face it, some things in life are unpredictable, and a nosebleed is one of them. Why does the nose suddenly decide to bleed? Is a nosebleed a sign of serious illness?

Most of the time, a nosebleed is nothing to worry about. Something as simple as a sneeze can cause one. So can low humidity. Without adequate moisture, sensitive nose membranes may dry and crack, opening tiny fissures. In addition, aging can thin nose membranes, making them vulnerable to rupture and bleeding. In some instances, however, a nosebleed can be a symptom of an underlying condition, such as high blood pressure, leukemia, liver disease, or a tumor.

SYMPTOMS

Symptoms of nosebleed include bright red blood if the bleeding occurs in the front of the nose; dark or bright red blood if the bleeding occurs in the back; light-headedness if there is a significant loss of blood; and shortness of breath or rapid heartbeat if there is a major loss of blood.

CAUSES

Causes of nosebleed include dry air, blowing the nose too hard, sinus infection, nasal infection, injury, a change in atmospheric pressure, an underlying condition (including high blood pressure, leukemia, liver disease, typhoid fever, malaria, hardening of the arteries, hemophilia, or a tumor), and the use of certain drugs (including aspirin, oral contraceptives, and anticlotting medications).

REMEDIES

- Sit down and tilt your head forward to prevent blood backup from gagging you.
- Pinch your nose for five minutes or more to dam and stop the bleeding.
- When the bleeding stops, do not blow your nose for at least 24 hours. You've got to allow time for a solid clot to form.
- If the bleeding does not stop quickly, pinch the fleshy part of the nose 10 minutes more and apply an ice pack to the bridge of the nose.

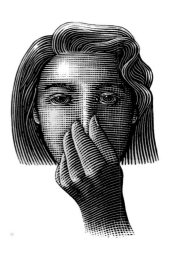

- If the bleeding has resulted from an injury, be gentle when you pinch the nose and be sure to apply ice.
- If the bleeding continues after 30 minutes, or if you are bleeding heavily, seek emergency treatment.
- To prevent nosebleeds, don't blow your nose like a trumpet. If you think a drug might be causing nosebleeds, ask your physician whether you can stop taking the drug or whether you can substitute another one.

Call your physician if your nosebleeds are frequent; your nosebleeds are hard to control; or you suspect a medication or an underlying illness such as high blood pressure could be causing your nosebleeds.

Sprains and Strains

It's the farm bowl, and it's your moment of glory. As you race through the potato field, the football tucked between chest and forearm, you elude tacklers with the grace of a gazelle. The result? A touchdown—and a pulled muscle.

Most of us have pulled up lame on occasion because of a strain or sprain suffered during a softball game, a tennis match, or even a romp in the yard with children.

A strain, or pulled muscle, occurs when a muscle stretches beyond its limits. In some cases, the muscle may tear or even rupture. If the strain results from sudden movement—a twist or a turn—you will experience severe pain at first, then tenderness and swelling. Bruises may appear after several days. If the strain results from overuse over a long period of time—that is, if it is chronic—you will experience soreness and tenderness several hours after the activity.

A sprain occurs when a ligament connecting a muscle to a bone tears. A tear may be mild or moderate, or it may be severe, causing a complete rupture. Sprains produce tenderness at first. Within hours, swelling, severe pain, black and blue discoloration, and limited mobility or disability occur.

Sprains and strains usually heal in two to four weeks. If the injury does not involve loss of mobility, it may not require a physician's treatment. Those sprains involving a rupture may require surgical treatment, however. When in doubt about the severity of an injury, call your physician.

CAUSES

Causes of strains and sprains include sudden twists and turns, overstretching, lifting, and bending.

SYMPTOMS

Pain, tenderness, swelling, stiffness, skin discoloration, and loss of mobility are symptoms of sprains and strains.

REMEDIES

- If you have a severely injured ankle, don't walk on it. Have someone help you from the scene. If you have a severe wrist or shoulder injury, have someone place your arm in a sling.

- Use the RICE treatment. RICE is an acronym for Rest, Ice, Compression, and Elevation.

Here's what to do:

1. Rest the injured part of the body.
2. Ice should be applied to the affected area.
3. Compress the injury with an elastic bandage or a cloth.
4. Elevate the injured part above the heart.

Continue applying ice to the injured area every two hours for 20 minutes to ease pain and reduce swelling. After 48 hours, you may substitute heat treatments. To apply heat, soak the injury in hot water or apply hot compresses. Keep the injured part elevated to allow fluid to drain, thereby reducing swelling. Use aspirin or ibuprofen to relieve pain.

Call your physician if your injury or your pain is severe or swelling and discoloration of the affected area continue to worsen even after treatment.

SORE THROAT

If your physician has diagnosed you with pharyngitis, don't worry. You needn't make out a will just yet. Pharyngitis simply means sore throat.

If your sore throat is the unfortunate result of postnasal drip or if it accompanies symptoms of the flu or a cold, then you can probably treat it yourself. Most sore throats clear up in two to six days.

CAUSES

There are many causes of sore throat, including bacterial, viral, and fungal infections; fatigue; allergies; smoking; postnasal drip; breathing through the mouth; air pollution; excessive coughing; and a variety of tooth and gum infections.

SYMPTOMS

Symptoms of sore throat include throat pain, swallowing difficulty, fever, swollen glands, appetite loss, headache, and red, swollen throat tissue.

REMEDIES

- Try gargling with salt water—1 teaspoon salt to a pint of water— or strong tea.
- Suck lozenges or hard candies throughout the day to help keep the throat moist.
- Drink plenty of fluids to lubricate the throat and prevent further irritation.
- Try eating raw garlic. Some studies indicate that garlic can help fight infection (see Medicine Chest, page 64).
- Use a cool-mist humidifier to help relieve dryness of the throat.

Call your physician if your sore throat is accompanied by a high fever, swollen glands, chills, fatigue, or pain that intensifies when you swallow.

SUNBURN

While at the beach, you're having so much fun swimming and waterskiing that you lose track of the time. Later, as you towel off and get ready for the trip home, you notice the burning, stinging pain all over.

"You look like a lobster," someone comments.

And you feel like a fool. After all, a sunburn, you're well aware, can put you at higher risk of developing skin cancer. Face it: You should have used a sunscreen. You should have limited your time in the sun.

But you didn't do either, and now your skin is red and swollen, and you're in pain. If the burn is severe enough to cause blistering, nausea, and vomiting, you should see a physician.

Next time, when outside in the sun, cover the skin with loose-fitting, light colored clothes made of loose-weave fabrics, and wear a hat. And don't forget sunscreen, available in oil, cream, paste, or liquid. It's probably best to use a sunscreen with a sun protection factor (SPF) of at least 15. Reapply your sunscreen frequently when out-of-doors.

Individuals who should be especially wary of the sun include those with a family history of skin cancer; those who burn easily; outdoor workers; pregnant women; and persons taking tranquilizers, diuretics, antihistamines, and antibiotics, all of which can increase the skin's sensitivity to the sun.

CAUSES

Sunburn is caused by overexposure to the ultraviolet rays of the sun, which are strongest between 10 AM and 3 PM. Sunlamps can also severely damage the skin.

SYMPTOMS

Symptoms of sunburn include pain, redness, swelling, and sometimes blistering of the skin; nausea and vomiting; chills; fever; and diarrhea.

REMEDIES

- Apply cool compresses to the affected area. When the compresses become warm, wet them again and re-apply. Continue the application for approximately 15 minutes. Repeat the procedure several times throughout the day.
- Take cool baths and drink plenty of water to restore fluids.
- If a blister is causing extreme pressure and discomfort, puncture it with a sterilized needle. But don't peel away the skin. Leave it in place; it protects the underlying skin against infection. Apply a skin cream containing aloe vera to the reddened skin around the blister.

Call your physician if your sunburn causes severe blistering; you experience nausea, vomiting, or diarrhea; your body temperature reaches 101 degrees or more; or pain and fever from sunburn continue for more than two days.

MEDICINE CHEST

RELIEVES

SCRATCHES
MINOR BURNS
SUNBURN

Today we have vaccines to protect ourselves from measles, chicken pox, and whooping cough. But if you grew up in the first half of this century, you may recall that these vaccines were not available—there were no instant cures.

On the second or third day of your illness, the doctor would show up at your door with his black bag bulging with the essentials of the healing art: a stethoscope, a "Say ah" stick, and a tiny hammer with which to strike your kneecaps. And let's not forget the variety of medicines he brought that could be swallowed or rubbed on.

Many of the following remedies may bring back childhood memories. Others may be new to you. Just remember, these remedies aren't meant to replace a doctor's care. So if you have suspicious or worrisome symptoms, give your doctor a call.

ALOE VERA

Farmers, lumberjacks, anglers, and hunters—all of whom get roughed up by everything from thorns and splinters to barbed wire and fish hooks—are among those who ought to keep aloe vera close by.

Aloe vera is a plant of the lily family native to Africa. Its secret lies in two ingredients: salicylates—the same anti-inflammatory agents found in aspirin—and magnesium lactate—an ingredient that inhibits skin reactions that cause itching. You can buy skin creams containing aloe vera at your local pharmacy. But you might find that aloe vera taken directly from the plant itself works best for treating minor skin damage.

Treatment: Buy an aloe vera plant at your local plant nursery or garden shop. Slit one of its leaves lengthwise, squeeze out the gel, and apply the gel directly to the injury site. Apply the gel five or six times a day until the affected area heals.

Warning: *Some people are allergic to aloe vera. If you develop a rash, stop using it.* ⚊ *Aloe vera has not been proven safe to treat indigestion, constipation, and other internal conditions.* ⚊ *Call your physician if you have a puncture wound or a serious burn.*

CHICKEN SOUP

Medical textbooks generally don't list chicken soup as a cold remedy. Nevertheless, it has been used for that purpose for many centuries—and to good effect.

The main benefit of chicken soup is that it helps clear congested nasal passages by promoting the flow of mucus. Besides helping to clear nasal passages, chicken soup also replenishes lost body fluids and helps to relieve throat pain and swelling.

Treatment: Use a recipe of your choice to make your chicken-soup remedy. (When making homemade soup, to lower the fat and cholesterol content, remove the chicken's skin before boiling. Make sure the chicken is thoroughly cooked before serv-

RELIEVES

COLDS & FLU

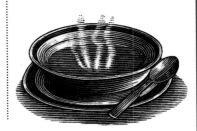

ing. Uncooked chicken may contain live salmonella bacteria, which can cause a serious infection of the digestive tract.) As the soup simmers, remember to keep the pot covered to prevent evaporation.

CRANBERRY JUICE

Cranberry juice not only prevents urinary tract infections, but it may cure them as well. How does it work? Some researchers believe the cranberry juice creates an acid in the urine that kills the bacteria that cause bladder infections. Others believe that an ingredient in cranberry juice prevents germs from clinging to the bladder walls.

Whether or not you believe in the cranberry cure, it still may be worth a try. At the very least, the juice will help you meet your daily requirement for vitamin C.

Treatment: Begin drinking cranberry juice at the first sign of a urinary-tract infection. If you've developed urinary-tract infections in the past, try drinking cranberry juice as a preventive measure. HINT: Because many cranberry juices available on store shelves contain high amounts of sugar, try taking cranberry juice in sugar-free tablet form.

Warning: *If you have the symptoms of a urinary tract infection, see your doctor. Besides drinking cranberry juice to help fight and cure the infection, you may need to take antibiotics as well.*

RELIEVES

URINARY TRACT
INFECTIONS

FEVERFEW

If you suffer from debilitating migraines, feverfew is the remedy you've been waiting for. Feverfew is an herb well known for its ability to fight migraine headaches. Apparently the herb inhibits blood-vessel dilation, a factor that plays a major role in causing migraines.

Fortunately, you can grow your own feverfew at home—indoors or out. For best results, sow the feverfew seedlings in late spring. Preparations are derived from the herb's leaves and flowers.

Treatment: For migraine control, chew two fresh (or frozen) feverfew leaves a day, or take a capsule containing 85 milligrams of leaf material. Feverfew is quite bitter. Most people prefer the capsules to chewing the leaves.

If feverfew capsules do not provide relief after a few weeks, don't give up on the herb without first changing brands. A recent study showed some brands of feverfew capsules contain only trace amounts of the herb.

Warning: *Talk to your doctor before using feverfew for the treatment of migraine.* ⟶ *Do not take feverfew if you are using an anti-clotting medication such as warfarin.* ⟶ *Feverfew may cause sores inside the mouth. If it does, discontinue taking the herb.* ⟶ *If you are pregnant, do not use this herb without first consulting your doctor.*

RELIEVES

MIGRAINE

USED TO TREAT

COLDS & FLU
HIGH BLOOD
PRESSURE
HIGH CHOLESTEROL
LEVELS

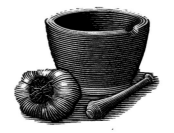

GARLIC

An herb of the lily family, garlic's healing reputation is almost as powerful as its smell. Not only does this wonder herb seem to prevent infection by the influenza virus, but garlic may work on the cold front, too.

Some research suggests that garlic may also reduce blood pressure and cholesterol levels and thin the blood, reducing the risk of developing blood clots. (Blood clots are a major cause of heart attacks and stroke.) In particular, there are two ingredients in garlic that produce this lifesaving, blood-thinning effect: adenosine and allicin.

Treatment: Adenosine remains effective even after cooking, according to studies by researchers at the University of Heidelberg in Germany. Allicin is effective only when garlic is eaten raw. So, if you're watching your heart's health, it's best to eat raw garlic—despite what your neighbors say.

To treat colds and flu, researchers recommend amounts of between 6 to 12 cloves of garlic a day. To help reduce blood pressure, cholesterol, and the likelihood of clots, 3 to 10 cloves of garlic a day are recommended.

Warning: *Talk to your doctor before taking higher than recommended doses of garlic.* ⌁ *Garlic causes stomach upset in some people.* ⌁ *If you are pregnant, do not use large amounts of this herb without first consulting your doctor.*

GINGER

Ever since ancient Asian sailors chewed ginger to quell their queasy stomachs, people have been using this remarkable spice to relieve stomach upset and nausea. So if your tummy is giving you trouble or you're suffering from a bout of motion sickness—give ginger a try.

Treatment: For motion sickness, the recommended dose is 1,500 milligrams in capsule form approximately 30 minutes before travel. (You can drink a 12-ounce glass of ginger ale instead, but it will be less effective against more intense symptoms.)

To relieve mild stomach distress, drink ginger ale or use ginger tea. To make ginger tea, use 2 teaspoons of powdered or grated ginger root per cup of boiling water. Steep 10 minutes before drinking.

Warning: *If you are pregnant, do not use this herb without first consulting your doctor.* ⚊ *Ginger has been shown to cause heartburn in some people.*

RELIEVES

MOTION SICKNESS
UPSET STOMACH

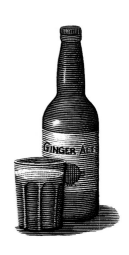

MINERAL OIL

Mineral oil is an excellent remedy for relieving dry skin and psoriasis, a disorder that causes red, scaly, itching skin patches that occur on the arms, ears, scalp, and pubic area.

For psoriasis sufferers, one of the advantages of mineral oil—besides the fact that it is an inexpensive substitute for costly moisturizers—is that it is pure, containing no additives or perfumes that could further irritate the skin.

Treatment: For psoriasis sufferers, the National Psoriasis Foundation recommends that you bathe first to moisten the skin. The mineral oil should be applied afterward, acting as a sealant to lock in the moisture. To treat simple dry-skin problems, apply mineral oil directly to affected areas as needed.

Warning: *Although some dictionaries define mineral oil as a laxative, most doctors frown on using it to relieve constipation because it interferes with the body's absorption of vitamins. If you take mineral oil as a laxative, follow your physician's instructions exactly.*

PARSLEY

If you'd like to try a natural remedy for bad breath, chew some parsley. The chlorophyll it contains, once digested, will sweeten the air you exhale, making you a pleasure to be around. Chlorophyll is the active ingredient in many commercial breath fresheners.

No, parsley won't cure bad breath, but it will help mask it. So, if you don't like commercial mouthwashes, it makes good "scents" to try this perennial herb.

Treatment: To freshen breath, eating a few sprigs of parsley will usually suffice.

USED TO TREAT

BAD BREATH

Warning: *High doses of parsley oil have been shown to cause headache, nausea, vertigo, hives, and liver and kidney damage.* ⟶ *If you are pregnant, do not take parsley without first consulting your doctor.*

PEPPERMINT

Menthol, the oil distilled from peppermint and other mints, is used to flavor beverages, desserts, candy, chewing gum, and medicine. The U.S. Food and Drug Administration has approved menthol as an active ingredient for several over-the-counter indigestion remedies as well because of the mint's ability to relax stomach muscles, enabling you to digest a meal with ease. So, for occasional indigestion, you might want to give peppermint tea a try.

Treatment: Boil one or two teaspoons of dried or fresh, crushed peppermint leaves to make peppermint tea. Drink a cup of the tea two or three times a day to help relieve the symptoms of indigestion.

Warning: *Avoid taking peppermint if you suffer frequent bouts of heartburn. Peppermint relaxes the stomach muscles, which could allow backup of stomach contents.* ⟶ *Do not give peppermint to babies or small children. The menthol in the tea may cause a choking sensation.* ⟶ *Do not take peppermint if you are breast-feeding; peppermint can reduce milk flow.*

USED TO TREAT

INDIGESTION

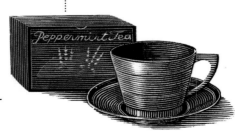

USED TO TREAT

POISONING

SYRUP OF IPECAC

Your medicine chest isn't complete if it doesn't contain syrup of ipecac. This remedy is used to induce vomiting in persons who have swallowed a non-caustic poison.

Before using syrup of ipecac, call an ambulance and call your local poison-control center (usually based at a hospital) for emergency assistance. Report the type of poison ingested, if known, and any other information the control center requests. If the control center advises using syrup of ipecac—for example, to bring up drugs or poisonous plants—then proceed with treatment.

Syrup of ipecac should not be used for all poisoning emergencies. In particular, you should not induce vomiting with syrup of ipecac, or any other remedy, if the patient is unconscious; you don't know what kind of poison the patient swallowed; or the patient has swallowed a caustic poison. Caustic poisons—such as lye, bleach, paint thinner, turpentine, and gasoline—burn when they are swallowed. Forcing the patient to vomit a caustic poison could seriously damage tissue when the poison comes back up.

Treatment: Give children one tablespoon of syrup of ipecac and adults two tablespoons. Children should drink half a glass of water afterward, and adults should drink a full glass of water or more. Vomiting should occur within 20 minutes. If it doesn't, repeat the dosage.

Individuals who are conscious and who have swallowed a caustic poison should be given milk, water, or milk of magnesia (a tablespoon in a cup of water) to dilute the poison. Seek medical attention immediately.

Warning: *If you suspect poisoning, call your local poison-control center immediately.*

TEA BAG

To rid yourself of those tiny ulcerations of the mouth called canker sores, grab a tea bag. Tea contains an astringent called tannic acid, which causes skin cells to shrink.

Treatment: To obtain relief from the pain of canker sores, apply the wet tea bag directly to the canker sore and hold in place for a few minutes.

YARROW POULTICE

The yarrow herb can be found in pastures and along roadsides throughout the northern hemisphere. Native Americans and pioneers applied it to minor skin cuts and abrasions to help fight infection.

Treatment: Yarrow can be used to promote healing in several ways. To make a poultice, bring water to a boil and pour the boiling water over the yarrow flowers, completely immersing them. Place the flowers in a strainer to drain excess water. Wrap the flowers in gauze and apply the poultice to the affected area. (Do

RELIEVES

CUTS & ABRASIONS

not apply yarrow to unwashed cuts. Because yarrow works fast, it will stop the bleeding while sealing in dirt.) After the bleeding subsides, remove the poultice and apply a bandage.

You can also place ground-up yarrow tips in a cup of hot water. Mix in glycerin, boric acid, and oil of wintergreen (a few teaspoons of each). Apply the resulting semi-liquid mixture to the injury site and wrap it in gauze.

A third option is to sprinkle yarrow powder on the cut. You can buy yarrow powder at natural-food stores.

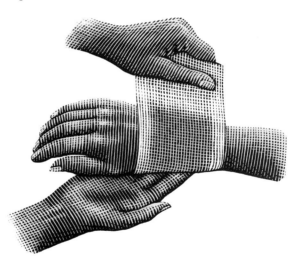

Warning: *Do not ingest yarrow. The herb is meant to be used as a topical application only.* — *If you are pregnant, do not use this herb without first consulting your doctor.*

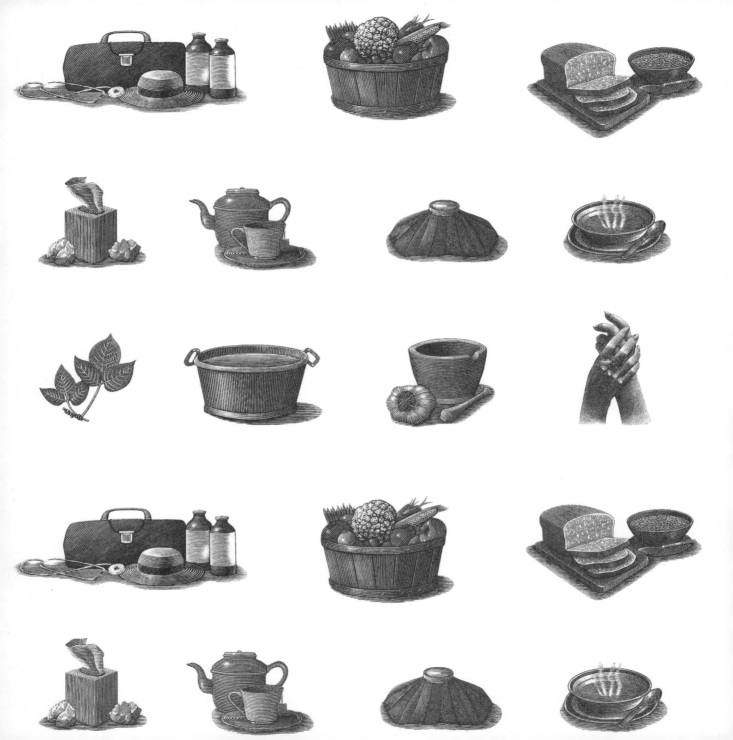